JUICING FOR WEIGHT LOSS NEWBIES

Over 50 Delicious Juicing Recipes That Enable You Loss Weight Naturally Fast, Increase Strength and Stamina

Morgan Green

<u>TABLE OF CONTENT</u>

Introduction......................4

Chapter one: Effectiveness of fruit and veggie juice recipes...12

Juicing recipe for body cleanse 12

Slimming Apple plum juice recipe 22

Carrot and Cucumber juice ...26

The Veggie detox juice 29

Fat burning Apple carrot juice with Celery 35

Pumpkin pie juice...................39

Chapter two: The Unique Green Juice Recipes..............................52

Green Juice 52

Super Cleanser 57

Citrus Veggie Green Juice 65

Apple and Fennel Mango Green Juice 68

Introduction

Thank you so much for taking out time to purchasing this book that helps you discover unique ways towards achieving the fastest ways to lose weight naturally including an increase in energy to enable you feel great.

We are thrilled to keep you informed about the essence of mother-nature and a whole lot of benefits through this practice as you go through it carefully.

Having yourself the benefits of acquiring these amazing collections of juicing recipes will aid you through every step to providing you with an amount of full scale of vitamins, nutrients, minerals and a lot more of micro-elements and burning all excess

weight naturally like you never ought to believe.

I will explain how it works but before I do so, make sure to place your mindset ready and serious to go through this very guide carefully.

The effectiveness and efficiency of Juicing is no miracle as much as it is no magic of a trick in cooking. It is categorically defined as a process of extraction (squeezing the juice) from fine vegetables or fruits. We can't deny or shy from the fact that it has become a current buzzword, but do you think or feel that it is easy to extracts the crowd's attention for no peculiar reason? You know the response to that question.

In essence, the very reason(s) why most people embark on juicing is of it positive benefits that are peculiar to a large amount of people who have passed through this practice and reaped it success in their body system.

Benefits of Juicing

The end result of vegetables is wealthy in nutrients: they're first-rate assets of vitamins, minerals, and antioxidants that the frame wishes to function well.

The juice extracted from sparkling fruits and vegetables incorporates the maximum of those nutrients, excluding the fiber and the antioxidants connected to fiber.

Small-scale research has suggested there are fitness blessings to ingesting clean juices.

Fruit and vegetable juices may additionally help delay the onset of Alzheimer's sickness, specifically amongst the ones at a higher chance of the ailment, a have a look at located.

In a small-scale experiment on wholesome person individuals, the extraordinary consumption of vegetable juice for three days appeared to adjust the intestine bacteria associated with weight loss. The contributors' frame weight and body mass index reduced, while their trendy properly-being increased.

Pomegranate juice, known to be a coronary heart-healthful juice, has been linked to the lower of ailment-contributing elements in patients with carotid artery stenosis (narrowing neck arteries). It has additionally shown promising results on sufferers with prostate cancer, prolonging PSA doubling time, as a consequence probably improving disorder effects. Pomegranate juice also progress insulin resistance amongst sufferers with kind-2 diabetes.

Apple juice, meanwhile, regarded to contribute to decreased danger of the form of coronary heart disease known as coronary artery disease.

Smooth consumption of certainly one of your five each day portions of greens

150 ml of juice counts as one among your 5 endorsed servings.

Sparkling juice can be finest for people with dental troubles or people who actually dread chewing fruits and greens. If munching on stalks of celery isn't your idea of amusing, consuming their juice makes it less difficult in an effort to still get some of the vitamins.

Juice also is available on hand while your morning routine doesn't permit time to enjoy platefuls of salad. You can make juice in bulk and keep it chilled as a quick, healthy drink for the times when your schedule is packed. Maximum juices may be stored inside the refrigerator for 2 or three days.

Because the juice is liquid, it gets absorbed lots faster by way of the frame than whole produce. This makes it a convenient pre- and publish-workout drink. it could supply your body the hydration and vitamins it desires to boost your overall performance without placing stress for your digestive machine.

Notice that all the juice you drink can most effectively ever count number as one component. You continue to need to virtually get the alternative 4 from whole produce.

Chapter one: Effectiveness of fruit and veggie juice recipes

Juicing recipe for body cleanse

Ultimate green Juice:

I drink this juice day by day, and with a suitable motive. the base is celery, that's a touch acknowledged nutritional powerhouse. It's loaded with potassium, folic acid, magnesium, calcium, iron, phosphorus, and important amino acids. On pinnacle of all that, it's one of the maximum alkalinizing matters you could put in your body. To the celery, I upload kale, green apple, parsley, lime, lemon, and ginger, creating an extremely strong, detoxifying cocktail.

Ingredients:

1 bunch celery

4-5 kale leaves (preferably lacinato)

1 inexperienced apple

One big handful of flat leaf parsley leaves

1 lime

1 lemon

1 inch of fresh ginger

Add one tablespoon of organic Coconut Oil for added health benefits.

Beet Apple and Blackberry Juice

Beet juice is a powerful cleanser of the blood, and pretty nutritious. It's full of foliate, manganese potassium, iron and nutrition C. To the beets, I upload apples, blackberries, and ginger, growing a deep pink and delicious elixir.

Beet Apple Blackberry Juice:

Beet Apple and Blackberry Juice photo via Shutter stock

Ingredients:

Three small beets

2-three apples

8 oz... Blackberries

Half inch fresh ginger

Picture by means of meals Thinkers

Wild Spiced Dandelion Berry Bliss Juice

This Wild highly spiced Dandelion Berry Bliss Juice is a first-rate instance of the way a pulped juice isn't always handiest healthier and more useful, it's far actually more texturally beautiful.

Wild Spiced Berry Juice:

Wild Spiced Berry Juice via Shutter stock

Components:

2 cups strawberries

1 cup dandelion leaves or extra to taste

1 cup raspberries

1 small chili with seeds and placental skin removed (greater or less depending on the heat) *non-obligatory

10-20 drops of alcohol-unfastened liquid stevia relying upon the ripeness and beauty of your berries *optional

Tropical paradise juice:

An appropriate manner to decorate your morning, this juice mixture is simple on the digestive gadget and gently loosens any building up that could have taken place even as the body became at relaxation.

Components:

1 medium ripe papaya, peeled, seeded, and sliced

1 small pineapple, peeled, cored, and sliced

1 (1-in.) piece peeled sparkling ginger

1 medium kiwi, peeled

1.2 cup sparkling young coconut water (stir in after juicing)

Juicy reality:

This juice changed into a danger discovery at a roadside juice stand at the lovely island of Kauai. Although the juice stand is not in an enterprise, we're satisfied to proportion this recipe and maintain this great-selling juice alive. it's miles truly super.

Blossoming lotus juice aide:

The simple components of this sparkling inexperienced juice create an uncommon combination. This candy, an herbal drink is a tremendous departure from mundane juice blends.

Blossoming Lotus Juice

Green juice image through Shutter stock

Elements:

Five huge Fuji apples, cored

1 (2-in.) piece peeled and sliced sparkling ginger

1 medium lime, outer 20 medium-huge sparkling rinds eliminated, white basil leaves pith intact

7 large sprigs cilantro sectioned

Juicy fact:

This juice is served in Oregon's Blossoming Lotus restaurant, co-owned by using our very own Bo Rinaldi. That is an all-time favorite signature providing inside the eating place and is respected for its Thai-stimulated flavors.

Lawn inexperienced Coconut Detox Juice:

Inexperienced Coconut Juice image thru Shutter stock

Garden green Coco

Coconuts are filled with potassium and electrolytes, says Helms, which makes them first-rate post-exercising drinks, and best for summer.

Components:

1 younger Thai coconut

1 handful of inexperienced kale

1 handful of spinach

½ bananas

Instructions:

Crack open coconut (the usage of a cleaver and intense care) and pour the coconut water into a blender. Take away coconut meat with a spoon and add to blender. Upload kale, spinach, and banana. Pour smoothie into the coconut and serve with a straw.

Spice-c juice:

Ingredients:

1 quarter sparkling pineapple

1 orange

1/2 handful cilantro

Half small jalapeno, seeded.

Slimming Apple plum juice recipe

If you need to make sure that your body is getting all the vitamins, nutrients, and minerals it wishes, juicing can be one of the best picks you could make in your fitness. so that you can get the equal quantity of vitamins from complete fruit, you'll consume more than is physically feasible for nearly any grownup to eat.

Beginning your day with wholesome, self-made juice does greater than provide your body the gas it needs to get through the day. It may additionally help you lose weight. In particular, plum and apple juice are each excellent at putting off belly fats in supporting you slender down. Do this recipe in your juicer.

Lose weight with Plums and Apples

Plums and apples have long been identified for his or her capability to aid weight reduction, help you feel complete, and preserve your digestive machine normal. Each culmination is high in fiber, so you can hold your digestive system transferring frequently and avoid the accumulation of stool for your device, which can make you appear bloated and puffy.

Furthermore, a huge glass of plum and apple juice may make it less difficult which will avoid cravings all day long. Those fruits are full of herbal sweeteners so that they should satisfy your candy enamel. This may provide you with a bit more strength of will whilst 2:00 rolls around and also you want to get a candy bar from the merchandising gadget.

Juice Recipe

So long as you have got a juicer, you are to your manner to some of the first-class-tasting plum and apple juice you have got ever had. There are numerous forms of plums available on the market nowadays. Pick out one with the extent of sweetness that suits your taste; this can encourage you to drink extra and preserve you away from introduced sweeteners.

This can consist of washing, peeling, and cutting. Of direction, don't forget about to take the pits out of the plums!

3 plums

1 cucumber

Half of apple

1/8 lemon

Put these elements into your juicer and revel in the stunning, delicious juice that comes out. I recommend consuming this first issue in the morning, as it can kick start your metabolism and assist your frame to burn fat more effectively all day lengthy.

Carrot and Cucumber juice

Would you adore undertaking a brand new wholesome addiction and beginning your day with a big glass of inexperienced juice to detoxify your frame, have extra energy during the day and get a flatter stomach? This cleansing Cucumber Carrot Juice is best for anybody who isn't conversant in the sturdy taste of leafy veggies yet but who nonetheless needs the equal cleansing impact. it is a super hydrating and barely sweet way to the carrots. Plus: it has a magic detox component that offers it a deep yellow shade… Curcumin!

Curcumin, often known as "the queen of spices", has very effective fitness advantages: it'll deeply cleanse your liver, raise your immune system & metabolism, reduce inflammation and help your body to save you healthy cells from turning into cancer cells. Curcumin has a strong, barely sour flavor so that you don't need tons.

Cleansing Cucumber Carrot Juice

SERVES: 1 individual (1 huge glass)

Equipment: juicer OR blender + nut milk bag/cheesecloth

Ingredients:

2 handfuls of chards

3 huge candy carrots

1 small cucumber

½ small lemons

1 tablespoon of ginger

1/eight teaspoon of turmeric powder

Directions:

Upload chards, carrots, cucumber, lemon, and ginger to the juicer. Pour into a tumbler.

Add the turmeric powder and stir nicely with a spoon.

The Veggie detox juice

Ingesting homemade clean juice is one of the simplest methods to enhance your immune device. Regardless of what form of juice it's miles, as long as its miles freshly made your body will advantage from it.

The way to make detox inexperienced juice:

First, accumulate all of the substances and rinse them very well. Reduce them into smaller pieces just so they match via the juicer chute. I additionally take away the tough components from apples however this isn't always necessary.

Now you are prepared for juice. The juicing itself takes less than five mins and you must get almost 3 cups of juice.

What are the things needed to make detox green juice

You may want a juicer. There are several sorts available on the market. The quality one in relation to preserving the maximum vitamins for your juice is a gradual press juicer. I individually use the classic centrifugal juicer that is quicker and also cheaper.

Nutribullet will not flip your greens right into a juice. it'll just puree them so you will come to be with smoothie-like texture.

Green juice benefits:

Rich in antioxidants

Facilitates keep healthful skin

Correct for cleaning your body from toxins

What does detox juice do?

A detox juice facilitates your frame cleanse through getting rid of pollution. Now you don't want to be just drinking juices whilst you want to cleanse your frame. Just eating light, healthy food for a few days after days of feasting is virtually excellent for you.

Many human beings drink juices simplest to lose weight or detox for several days. I rather propose consulting a specialist before doing this.

Strive including this detox inexperienced juice in your food regimen that consists of slight portions of protein, veggies, the end result, wholesome fats, and complete grains.

You can also start with drinking frame cleansing Lemon Ginger Water each morning, in case you don't have a juicer. If you do, I've additionally sparkling skin inexperienced Juice Recipe on my blog that is also amazing if you need to hold healthful.

How do you make the best-inexperienced juice?

I without a doubt believe that there may be no right or wrong in terms of making green juice or any sort of juice for that rely on. To me, the exceptional juice is the one you want. Consequently, I propose you experiment with the elements if you experience find it irresistible is not for your liking the primary time.

The key to creating the fine juice is to locate more of the culmination or veggies you adore and use much less of those you don't. Whilst attempting a new recipe for the primary time I endorse sticking to the recipe. Then flavor it. In case you are not happy with its flavor add greater lemon, maybe a touch of maple syrup or more apples, cucumber, grapes … the alternatives are countless.

Tips for making and drinking detox inexperienced juice:

Self-made juices are first-class enjoyed properly after juicing. However, if saved properly they can be stored in the fridge for up to forty-eight hours.

Shop it in a tumbler jar/bottle sealed with a lid.

This juice is full of nutrients (A, B, C, E, okay), Manganese, Iron, Potassium, and other minerals. Including it for your diet and consuming reasonably will not simplest help your body cleanse however also boosts your immune system and maintains healthful pores and skin.

Bear in mind: detoxifying your body is ideal however doing change juice for a meal. Alternatively, upload it to your meal.

Continually seek advice from a consultant if you need to do a juice detox only. They'll propose you what is pleasant for you.

Fat burning Apple carrot juice with Celery

Apple Carrot Celery Juice is effective as a weight reduction resource for 2 vital reasons.

One reason that it's so powerful is Actual for all juicing recipes; sparkling fruit and vegetable liquids are very low in calories, notably filling, and extremely nutritious.

The alternative component that makes this specific veggie combo an excellent one while using a juicer for weight reduction lies inside the potassium and sodium ratio within the celery.

Celery has a stability of sodium and potassium that works to truly stimulate urine and assist take away extra water and uric acid from the kidneys. In case you are juicing to drop extra kilos, you may accurately accelerate the loss of water weight in a natural manner by adding celery on your beverages.

Additional fitness blessings of this juicing recipe:

• Carrots are very excessive in vitamin A, as well as nutrients B and C, Iron, and Calcium.

• Apples are excessive in vitamins and minerals and are a terrific supply of pectin and antioxidants.

• Celery has a compound called Phthalide, which can reduce excessive blood pressure by enjoyable the vessels that blood flows through.

• Without adding any huge energy on your each day consumption, you get a beneficiant dose of an extensive collection of very valuable nutrients and minerals.

3 Carrots

½ Cucumbers

1 Apple

2 Celery sticks

Wash all fruits and greens properly. Reduce the ends off of the carrots before juicing them. It's now not vital to peel or deseed any of the fruit or veggies; the juicer will separate it for you. Drink the mixture at once after you make it for the very best nutritional value.

Juicing fruits and veggies is extremely wholesome. There isn't always an unmarried bottled emblem obtainable that could even come near competing with what fresh juice has to provide. Aside from being greater healthy, some mass-produced juices are actually dangerous because of their delivered preservatives and sugars. Whilst you make your personal at home, it's now not the most effective sparkling, it's additionally 100% natural.

Pumpkin pie juice

If you're new to juicing, the idea may additionally sound a chunk unappealing to you. Nobody is eating raw pumpkin, let alone ingesting focused juice, right?

And but all of the juicing aficionados know they have in their recipe books at least some properly-worn pages in which the pumpkin juice recipes are.

On this put up, you may research 5 smooth recipes to make the tastiest and healthiest juices and milkshakes from the pumpkin.

The bright orange color of pumpkin suggests that it is a rich source of nutrition A and beta-carotene. And actually it's miles!

As soon as an ounce of raw pumpkin includes a hundred and seventy% of your day by day need of nutrition A. uncooked pumpkin juice is naturally loaded with the nutrition, making it really one of the excellent liquids to your eyes.

The nutrition- A in pumpkin juice now not simplest enables with keeping and improving your imaginative and prescient, but your pores and skin too.

Apart from the pre-nutrition A with a view to being changed into retinol in the body, pumpkin juice has a small quantity of a compound that is equivalent to retinol, which is famous for its anti-getting old consequences on the skin.

The juice also includes a high amount of numerous antioxidants, consisting of nutrition C and zinc. These are vital for a healthy, easy, acne-unfastened pores and skin!

Pumpkin juice is a quite secure drink, besides to individuals who are allergic to pumpkin. The handiest side-impact acknowledged to us is that it may turn your skin orange or yellow. However, that simplest takes place in case you eat a large quantity of it each day over a long duration, which most of the people don't.

A way to prepare a pumpkin for juicing

Choose a small/common pumpkin, the sort that you can make a pie with. Pumpkins that experience heavy for his or her sizes and have smooth skin are the quality.

Wash the pumpkin very well and do away with the stem.

Reduce the pumpkin into halves. it can be very difficult

Scoop out the seeds and the stringy pulp.

Peel the pumpkin and cut it into small chunks that could undergo your juicer.

Fine pumpkin juice recipes:

Those are very clean juice and smoothie recipes with pumpkin. a number of them don't even require a juicer to make!

1. PUMPKIN CARROT JUICE (three SERVINGS)

The Juice

With pumpkin and carrot, this juice is complete of diet A and C. A amazing treat to your eyes and skin!

Tips:

You could also pour the juice into a hermetic jar and put in into the fridge for a few hours before ingesting it. It tastes higher whilst cold.

Elements:

1 small pumpkin

Three medium carrots

1 medium apple

½ inch ginger root

½ teaspoon cinnamon powder

The way to make:

Prepare the pumpkin as directed above

 Wash and peel the carrots, put off the stem, and reduce into chunks that healthy on your juicer

Wash and peel the ginger.

Run the whole thing through your juicer.

Add the cinnamon powder, stir properly, and revel in.

PUMPKIN CARROT JUICE (five SERVINGS)

The Juice

This is a thick, delicious juice that doesn't incorporate too much energy. Pumpkin and apple ciders are each incredible supply of nutrition C and diverse antioxidants that assist stabilize blood sugar and kill pathogens.

Substances:

- 4 cups (950ml) apple cider

- 6 tablespoons pumpkin puree

- 1¼ cup peach nectar

- ¼ teaspoon floor cinnamon (non-compulsory)

How to make:

Pour the content to a blender. add the cinnamon powder.

Close the blender and run it until the substances are all blended.

Pour the juice into a hermetic jar and go away it in the fridge to sit back.

Serve the juice cold. If it's too thick, you could also serve it with ice.

Pumpkin apple juice (5 servings):

The Juice

An easy-to-make juice with wonderful flavor from apple, pumpkin, and peach,

Pumpkin apple juice recipe

Elements:

2 cups of water

12 oz (350 ml) apple juice concentrates. You may make your very own apple juice by means of going for walks cored apples via a juicer.

15 oz (450 ml) pumpkin puree

1 cup frozen sliced peaches

A way to make:

Add the frozen peach into the water, and go away it there for a few minutes to allow it thaw.

Use a blender to pulse the peach and the water.

Upload the apple juice listen, the pumpkin, and the lemon juice. Run the blender till the entirety is well blended.

Strain the combination using cheesecloth or a nut milk bag.

Pour the juice into a tumbler jar and go away it inside the refrigerator for some hours. This juice is pretty skinny; therefore, its fine served cold without ice.

Pumpkin apple cider juice (5 servings):

The Juice

With honey and ginger, this pumpkin juice offers a splendid enhance in your immune and digestive system.

Pumpkin apple juice

Ingredients:

Five cups apple cider

2 inches sparkling ginger, sliced

1 cinnamon stick

½ teaspoon entire cloves

¼ cup honey

½ cup brown sugar

1 (28-ounce) can pumpkin puree

A way to make:

Heat 3 cups apple ciders in a saucepan add ginger, cinnamon, and cloves.

Boil the combination. Simmer for approximately 15mins.

Stir in honey and sugar. Transfer to an included glass field and go away in the refrigerator to chill.

When serving, stir in 2 cups apple cider and pumpkin puree. First-rate enjoy when bloodless.

5. Pumpkin banana milkshake (2 servings)

The Juice

Full of protein, vitamins, and minerals along with calcium, potassium, phosphorus, and magnesium, this milkshake is a notable snack to begin your day with!

Components:

1 frozen banana

½ cup (120 g) vanilla Greek yogurt

¼ teaspoon cinnamon powder

¼ teaspoon pumpkin pie spice

½ cup (one hundred twenty ml) skim milk

Two spoon-full of pure maple syrup

⅔ Cup (150g) pumpkin puree

Whipped cream for topping

A way to make:

Upload everything into a blender within the indexed order.

Run the blender for three minutes or till the combination is easy. Upload extra ice or more milk if desired.

Leave inside the fridge till nicely-chilled. Pour the mixture into a glass, and pinnacle with whipped cream. Serve cold.

Chapter two: The Unique Green Juice Recipes

Green Juice

Green juice is categorized as a beverage crafted from the juices of green veggies.

There's no reliable recipe, but common elements include celery, kale, Swiss chard, spinach, wheatgrass, cucumber, parsley, and mint.

For the reason that inexperienced juice has a tendency to taste bitter, most recipes upload small quantities of fruit which may or won't be green to sweeten it and improve its normal palatability. Famous fruit options consist of apples, berries, kiwi, lemons, oranges, and grapefruit.

The maximum dedicated inexperienced juice drinkers prefer fresh, homemade juice; however, you could buy it from specialty juice cafés too.

Business inexperienced juices are to be had as well, but a few sorts comprise introduced sugar, which reduces the drink's nutrient density. Extra sugar consumption is likewise related to numerous damaging health outcomes.

Moreover, many bottled inexperienced juices are pasteurized. This method heats the juice to kill harmful micro organism and enlarge shelf existence, but it is able to damage some of the warmth-touchy nutrients and plant compounds located in clean juice

Green juice is not an alternative choice to a balanced and healthful weight-reduction plan, but it stocks some of the benefits that come in conjunction with consuming greater end result and vegetables.

Green vegetables and their juices are extraordinary resources of numerous important vitamins, minerals, and beneficial plant compounds. As an example, Swiss chard and kale are filled with vitamins A and ok, whilst wheatgrass materials masses of nutrition C and iron

Studies suggest that ingesting leafy inexperienced greens every day may additionally assist lessen irritation, heart sickness danger, and your threat of age-associated intellectual decline.

There's also proof that certain compounds in clean juice can function as prebiotics, which feeds and aid the boom of useful micro organisms living on your digestive tract.

Recurring periodic intake is related to numerous blessings, such as reduced constipation, weight maintenance, and improved immune function.

Furthermore, many human beings locate that consuming their veggies and fruits is an easy and efficient way to reinforce their consumption of treasured vitamins.

Eventually, sure humans, such as folks that had a surgical operation at the belly or intestines, can benefit from inexperienced juice, as it's less difficult to digest. For those populations, juicing is a quick-time period option for the duration of recovery.

Speak on your healthcare company or dietitian about juicing on your precise circumstance.

Super Cleanser

The Grasp Cleanse also called the master cleanser or the lemonade food plan is a brief-term liquid food plan this is famous for individuals who need to lose weight quickly or reset their diets in the direction of healthier consuming. Folks who cross at the food regimen drink a lemon beverage and saltwater for at least 10 days to slim down. Like maximum liquid fasts, this system isn't always supported by using the mainstream medical or nutrition community.

How it Works

The Master Cleanse is a liquid weight loss program. It includes consuming a gallon of saltwater and six to 12 glasses of a lemonade concoction a day. The full daily consumption is more or less equivalent to the juice of three to six lemons in step with day, which includes some important vitamins. it also carries .75 to 1.five cups of maple syrup per day.

Apart from the lemonade drink, herbal laxative teas are endorsed as part of each day routine. Colonics and enemas aren't commonly recommended at the master Cleanse.

What to devour

The main focus of the Master Cleanse is homemade lemonade that contains lemon juice, maple syrup, water, and a touch cayenne pepper.

Compliant meals:

Unique-recipe lemonade

Saltwater

Senna-primarily based natural tea

Non-Compliant ingredients:

All different meals

Lemons and maple syrup are used due to the fact they're without problems available and are a rich supply of vitamins and minerals. Lemons are also considered a cleaning, healing meal in alternative medicine. Three at the same time as lemon juice and maple syrup do incorporate some nutrients and minerals, many different meals have the same quantity or more of vitamins and minerals.

As an example, one of the touted advantages of the lemons is potassium; however one banana incorporates about the same quantity of potassium as all the lemon juice consumed each day on the Grasp Cleanse.

Endorsed Timing

The grasp Cleanse recommends starting every day with a saltwater flush, then consuming several cups of the lemonade during the day, and finishing the day by means of consuming a cup of a laxative, senna-primarily based herbal tea. The eating regimen is recommended for at least 10 days and most of forty days. According to the ebook, people can repeat the grasp Cleanse 3 to 4 times a year.

After cleanse is over, a breaking rapid protocol is usually recommended. The primary day after cleanse, the handiest orange juice is allowed. The second one day entails greater orange juice and probable vegetable soup. On day three, greens, salads, and fruit are allowed. Regular eating is commonly resumed on the fourth day.

Professionals and Cons

Like most fad diets, the grasp Cleanse has a mix of positives and negatives. For the reason that diet is composed handiest of drinking particularly mixed lemonade, it promises speedy weight reduction. But, no different meals are allowed on the plan, which calls for a high-quality deal of strength of mind to combat via starvation. Plus, while you may fast lose weight, you might gain it lower back simply as quickly once the short ends.

Professionals:

Brief weight loss

A religious or psychological raise

Cons:

Does now not offer adequate vitamins

No meals allowed

Weight reduction isn't sustained

May purpose gallstones

Pros:

The Master Cleanse is promoted as a brief weight loss rapid, and if you may stick with the plan, it'll supply. In keeping with the book, a weight reduction of two kilos consistent with day is standard.

Many testimonials on the net claim that the grasp Cleanse can lessen signs of persistent infection and pain, enhance power, and enhance intellectual clarity all through and after the cleanse. A few human beings record an uplifting spiritual or psychological impact, which may additionally have a tremendous impact on health.

Cons:

Most nutritionists and fitness specialists endorse against extended fasting (more than several days), specifically as a manner to shed pounds, due to the feasible fitness dangers.

One of the maximum not unusual worries is the shortage of vitamins, protein, and energy in the eating regimen.

Having six glasses of the lemonade beverage offers 650 or so calories a day, ensuing in a short weight loss. One of the capability side outcomes of rapid weight reduction in the formation of gallstones.6

Similarly, many people file feeling dizzy, faint, or extremely hungry at the grasp Cleanse and say the plan is hard. Loose stools and diarrhea are not unusual due specifically to the herbal laxative and saltwater drink. Frequent bowel actions are advocated on the eating regimen because they may be believed to resource in the elimination of pollutants.

Citrus Veggie Green Juice

Citrus inexperienced Juice consists of inexperienced veggies and citrus fruits for a slightly tart green juice. That is a simple green juice to make that still tastes exceptional.

Climate you are on cleanse or simply trying to stay healthy juicing is a great way to add more fruits & greens and their accompanying minerals & nutrients into your food plan.

Equipment you will need:

Juicer

Peeler

Cutting Board

Knife

Elements

Four leaves of kale

1 cucumber

1 small inexperienced apple

1 orange

1 lemon

Half lime

Instructions

Rinse kale and apple.

Peel cucumber, orange, lemon & lime.

Reduce the whole thing in portions small sufficient to fit your juicer.

Juice all ingredients.

Pour into a tumbler and revel in.

Recipe Notes

You may maintain the pores and skin of the cucumber I advise most effective if it's miles organic.

Apple and Fennel Mango Green Juice

Fennel is famous for its licorice-like taste and health blessings. Mixing it collectively with apples, lemon juice, and martini effects in a high-quality drink that you may truly admire

This apple & fennel juice blends a conventional juicing fruit with a completely not going component into a smooth and fresh concoction. Ensure to use very young bulbs of fennel handiest, as they have got much less "chunk in" taste and feature a totally fruity taste. Relax the fruits nicely before juicing them.

Ingredients required

240 grams fennel bulb

2 apples

2 piece fennel stalk with leafs

Fennel leaves for decoration

Half of Lemon Juice

2 Martini glasses

A way to prepare the Apple & Fennel Juice

Reduce the fennel bulb in half of after which into wedges, getting rid of the tough stem element at the bottom of the bulb.

Slice the apple in wedges and force each fruit through a juicer.

Blend with the lemon juice to avoid discoloration and in line with taste, then garnish with the fennel stalk and the fennel sprigs and serve without delay.